I0536125

Table of Contents

1. Introduction

Welcome to "Chair Yoga for Seniors," a guide designed to bring the numerous benefits of yoga to individuals in their golden years. This chapter provides an overview of the book and sets the stage for your journey into the world of chair yoga.

The Benefits of Chair Yoga for Seniors

Aging gracefully involves maintaining physical and mental well-being. Chair yoga offers a gentle and accessible way for seniors to stay active, improve flexibility, build strength, enhance balance, and experience relaxation. From alleviating joint pain to boosting mood and reducing stress, chair yoga provides a holistic approach to health tailored to the needs of seniors.

How to Use This Book

In this chapter, you'll discover how to navigate the book effectively to maximize your chair yoga experience. Learn about the layout, the organization of chapters, and the importance of gradual progression. Whether you're new to yoga or a seasoned practitioner, understanding how to utilize this guide will ensure a comfortable and enriching journey through the practice of chair yoga.

As you embark on this path, keep in mind that chair yoga is not just about physical movements. It's about embracing mindfulness, connecting with your breath, and cultivating a positive relationship with your body. Throughout this book, you'll find detailed instructions, tips for safe practice, modifications for varying abilities, and insights into integrating chair yoga into your daily life.

So, let's begin this transformative journey together. The next chapter will delve into what chair yoga truly is and who stands to benefit from it. Prepare to experience the joy of movement, the tranquility of meditation, and the sense of well-being that chair yoga can bring to your life.

2. Understanding Chair Yoga

In this chapter, we'll delve deeper into the concept of chair yoga and explore its benefits, suitability for different individuals, and safety considerations. By understanding the foundations of chair yoga, you'll be better equipped to embrace its practice with confidence and enthusiasm.

What is Chair Yoga?

Chair yoga is a gentle form of yoga that adapts traditional yoga postures to be performed while seated or using a chair for support. It's an inclusive practice that caters to a wide range of physical abilities and mobility levels. The primary focus is on maintaining the mind-body connection through breath, movement, and meditation, even when mobility is limited.

Who Can Benefit from Chair Yoga?

Chair yoga is an excellent option for seniors, individuals with limited mobility, and those recovering from injuries. It's also suitable for anyone looking for a gentle and accessible introduction to yoga. The practice is not limited by age or physical condition, making it an inclusive choice for people at various stages of life.

Safety Considerations

Prioritizing safety is crucial in any exercise regimen, and chair yoga is no exception. This chapter will discuss essential safety considerations, such as avoiding overexertion, listening to your body, and understanding the limits of your own mobility. It will also provide guidance on seeking medical advice before starting a new exercise routine, especially if you have pre-existing health conditions.

Safety considerations for seniors before starting chair yoga exercises:

Consult a Healthcare Professional: Before seniors begin a new yoga practice, they should consult their doctor or healthcare provider, especially if they have any pre-existing health conditions or concerns.

- **Choose the Right Class:** Look for classes that are specifically designed for seniors or gentle yoga. These classes will emphasize safe and appropriate poses for older adults.
- **Start Slowly:** Seniors should begin with basic and gentle poses, gradually progressing to more advanced ones as their flexibility and strength improve.
- **Use Props:** Props such as blocks, straps, and blankets can provide support and stability during poses, making them more accessible for seniors.
- **Focus on Balance and Stability:** Incorporate poses that help improve

balance and stability, which can help prevent falls and injuries. Poses like Tree Pose, Warrior II, and Chair Pose can be beneficial.

- **Avoid Overstretching:** Seniors should avoid pushing themselves into deep stretches. Instead, they should focus on maintaining a comfortable stretch without pain.
- **Listen to Your Body:** Encourage seniors to pay attention to their body's signals. If a pose causes pain or discomfort, they should ease out of it or modify it accordingly.
- **Breathe Mindfully:** Breathing is an essential aspect of yoga. Seniors should focus on deep, mindful breaths throughout their practice, which can help relax the body and mind.
- **Warm-up and Cool-down:** Always start with a gentle warm-up to prepare the body for movement and

end with a cool-down to help the body relax and recover.

- **Stay Hydrated:** Seniors should drink water before, during, and after their yoga session to stay hydrated.
- **Modify Poses:** Many yoga poses can be modified to suit different levels of flexibility and ability. Seniors should feel comfortable making modifications that work for their bodies.
- **Avoid Inversions:** Some inversions, like headstands and shoulder stands, might not be suitable for all seniors due to the increased risk of injury. It's best to avoid these unless under the guidance of an experienced instructor.
- **Mind the Joints:** Seniors should be cautious with poses that place excessive pressure on the joints, especially the wrists and knees. Proper alignment is crucial to prevent strain.

- **Stay in Communication:** If attending a class, seniors should inform the instructor about any limitations or health concerns they have, so the instructor can provide appropriate guidance.
- **Rest and Recovery:** It's important to give the body adequate time to recover between yoga sessions. Seniors should not push themselves too hard and ensure they get enough rest.

Remember, safety is the top priority. Encourage seniors to listen to their bodies, practice patience, and enjoy the many benefits that yoga can offer in terms of flexibility, strength, and overall well-being.

By grasping these fundamental aspects of chair yoga, you'll be well-prepared to embark on your practice with confidence. The subsequent chapters will introduce you to practical aspects of chair yoga, including setting up your practice space, acquiring necessary props, and diving into foundational chair yoga poses. Remember, chair yoga is about embracing your body's unique abilities and discovering the joy of movement and mindfulness at your own pace.

3. Getting Started

As you embark on your chair yoga journey, it's important to set the stage for a comfortable and enjoyable practice. This chapter will guide you through the process of preparing your space, acquiring the necessary props, and ensuring that you have everything you need to make your chair yoga sessions a success.

Setting Up Your Space

Creating a peaceful and inviting space for your chair yoga practice is essential for cultivating a positive experience. Find a quiet and clutter-free area where you can practice without distractions. Arrange your chair on a stable surface, ensuring that it's positioned comfortably and that you have enough room to move around.

Necessary Props and Equipment

While chair yoga minimizes the need for props, having a few supportive items can enhance your practice. This chapter will introduce you to common props such as yoga blocks, straps, and blankets, which can provide added comfort and support during certain poses. You'll learn how to use these props effectively to adapt poses to your individual needs.

Attire and Comfort

Wearing comfortable clothing that allows for easy movement is key to a successful chair yoga practice. Choose clothing that allows you to stretch and breathe without restrictions. Additionally, you might consider having a small cushion or pillow on hand to further enhance your comfort during seated poses.

With your space set up and your props ready, you're well-prepared to embark on the practical aspects of chair yoga. The subsequent chapters will introduce you to foundational chair yoga poses that focus on gentle movements, flexibility, strength, and relaxation. Remember, chair yoga is about embracing your body's capabilities, nurturing your well-being, and finding a sense of balance and tranquility in each session.

4. Basic Chair Yoga Poses

Welcome to the practical heart of your chair yoga journey! This chapter introduces you to a variety of foundational chair yoga poses designed to gently stretch and mobilize your body. These poses are ideal for improving flexibility, enhancing circulation, and promoting relaxation. Remember, the key to chair yoga is not perfection in the poses, but rather a focus on how they make you feel.

Seated Mountain Pose

- Sit on a chair with your feet flat on the floor, hip-width apart.
- Lengthen your spine and relax your shoulders.
- Rest your hands on your thighs or by your sides.
- Engage your core muscles and gently tuck your chin.

- Inhale deeply, and as you exhale, imagine a string pulling the crown of your head toward the ceiling.
- Hold the pose for 5-10 breaths.

Seated Cat-Cow Stretch

This exercise increases spine flexibility and releases tension in the neck and shoulders.

- Sit comfortably on a chair with your feet flat on the floor.
- Place your hands on your knees.
- Inhale and arch your back, lifting your chest and gazing upward (Cow).
- Exhale and round your spine, tucking your chin toward your chest (Cat).
- Repeat the sequence 5-10 times, moving with your breath.

Gentle Neck and Shoulder Exercises

Begin with gentle neck movements and shoulder rolls to release tension and promote flexibility in these often-stressed areas. These exercises are particularly beneficial for those who spend long hours sitting or working at a computer.

Overhead Stretch

Begin in a seated position, facing forward with your arms down by your sides. Take a long, deep breath in and slowly stretch your arms upward to the ceiling. Hold this position for a moment, and bring your arms back downward with a long exhale. Throughout this exercise, make sure your core is engaged and your back is as straight as possible.

Neck Stretch

Sit up straight in your chair, and do not let your back touch the back of your chair. Extend your neck slowly upward so you feel the crown of your head rising towards the ceiling. While holding the base of your chair with your right hand, slowly reach upwards with your left hand to hold your left temple.

Take a deep breath, and upon exhalation, gently dip your left ear towards your left shoulder without bending your back or raising your right shoulder. Take several slow breaths in and out in this position, before alternating this stretch to the opposite side.

Reverse arm hold

Begin this pose in a seated position with your back straight and apart from the back of the chair. While you inhale deeply, reach your arms straight out to your sides at a low and wide angle. Exhale slowly and reach your hands behind your back, bending your elbows slightly. Arch your back slightly to feel the stretch in your shoulders, and take several breaths in and out.

Chair pigeon

Sit upright with your back away from the back of the chair and facing forward. Gently raise your left ankle to rest on top of your right knee or thigh. If you have trouble bringing your ankle to your knee, feel free to use your hand to assist. Inhale deeply, flex your left foot slightly, and bend forward upon exhale. After several deep breaths in the forward position, return to sitting up straight. Gently switch sides, so your right ankle is resting upon your left thigh or knee, and repeat the above steps.

Eagle arms

Sit upright in your chair and stretch your arms straight out in front of you. Cross your left arm over your right arm, and bend your elbows to bring your forearms together. Interlace your fingers and raise your elbows slightly, arching your back a bit. Hold this position for several deep breaths. Upon completion, switch to your right arm over your left arm.

Chair warrior

Begin this pose facing forward with your arms down by your side at a wide and low angle, or with one leg across the chair with your torso turned forward (if youre flexible enough for this position). Take a deep breath and slowly raise your arms straight above your head. Hold this pose for several breaths before lowering your arms back down to your sides. If you begin this pose with your leg across the chair, switch to the opposite leg across the chair and perform this pose again.

Side Bend

Begin by sitting upright, a little forward from the back of your chair, with your feet hip-width apart. Keep your right arm relaxed by your side, and inhale as you raise your left arm out and up toward your ear, palm facing inward. As you exhale, tilt your torso to the right. Do not over-extend only go as far as you are comfortable, and make sure your weight is balanced on both sides of your hips and glutes. Hold this position for three breaths. Inhale, reach your left arm to the sky, and recenter your torso. Continue to lower your arm as you exhale. Repeat on your right side, then continue until youve performed these movements three times on each side.

Arm Circles

Start by sitting upright near the edge of your chair, keeping your feet firmly on the ground. Put your left hand on your chest, then raise your right arm and move it in five circles forwards, then five circles backwards. Repeat these motions for your left arm, with your right hand resting on your chest.

This exercise is great for stimulating blood flow to the heart and for increasing strength and flexibility in the shoulders.

Bending the Legs

Sit at the front of your chair with your feet on the ground. Extend your right leg and lift it so your foot is in line with your hips, if possible. Then, put both your hands behind the right knee, interlock your fingers, and straighten your back as you inhale. On the exhale, simultaneously bend your right knee and bring your forehead toward it. Inhale and straighten your back and knee again and repeat the bending motion once more on the exhale. Do the same exercise on the left side. Complete three rounds of this exercise on each side.

This exercise activates the core, strengthens the hip and knee joints, and promotes flexibility.

Bicycles

Sit at the front of your chair and lean your shoulders back to rest on the back of the chair. Raise your right leg and make a pedaling motion, as if you are riding a bike.

Make this motion five times before resting your foot back on the floor. Repeat on the left side.

This is a good exercise for increasing strength in the abdomen and legs, as well as promoting circulation.

Spinal Twist

Sitting straight on the front of your chair, put your hands behind your head and link your fingers together. Inhale and stretch your elbows backwards as much as you feel comfortable. On the exhale, slowly twist your torso to the right and look toward your right elbow. Inhale and slowly turn back to the center. Repeat on the left side. Complete three rounds on both sides.

This exercise can help release tension in the upper back, neck, and shoulders, as well as promote flexibility in the spine

Tiger Breathing

Think of this exercise like a seated cat-cow pose. Sit near the front of your chair with your hands on your knees and your feet on the ground hip-width apart. As you inhale, tilt your hips forward and bend backwards, leaning your head back. On the exhale, do the opposite arch your back forward like a cat and tilt your hips backwards, bringing your chin down. Complete these movements four to eight times. Be sure to perform this exercise slowly and focus on your breathing.

As you practice these basic poses, pay close attention to your body's response. Breathe deeply and mindfully, honoring your limits and respecting any sensations you experience. Remember, chair yoga is about adapting the practice to your unique needs, so feel free to modify poses as necessary.

In the following chapters, you'll explore chair yoga for flexibility, strength, balance, and relaxation. Each pose you learn adds to the foundation of your practice, allowing you to build a customized routine that suits your goals and preferences. Enjoy the process of discovering how chair yoga can benefit your physical and mental well-being.

5. Chair Yoga for Flexibility

Flexibility is a cornerstone of well-being, allowing us to move freely and with ease. In this chapter, you'll delve into a series of chair yoga poses specifically designed to enhance your flexibility. These poses gently stretch and open different parts of your body, promoting suppleness and improving your range of motion.

Seated Forward Bends and Hamstring Stretches

This pose stretches the hamstrings and lower back, promoting relaxation.

- Sit on the edge of a chair with your feet hip-width apart.
- Inhale and lengthen your spine.
- Exhale and hinge at your hips, folding forward over your legs.
- Allow your hands to rest on your shins, ankles, or the floor.

Hip Opening Poses

Your hips play a vital role in your mobility and posture. Discover chair yoga poses that target the hip area, promoting flexibility and reducing stiffness. These movements can be particularly beneficial for individuals with hip discomfort or tightness.

Do these for hip openers exercise:

- **Butterfly Stretch:** Butterfly stretch is a seated hip opener that is gentle enough for all levels. To do it, sit on the floor with your spine long. Bend both knees so that you can bring the soles of your feet together. Stay right here, or reach your hands around your feet as you hinge at your hips and fold, bringing your torso over your legs. You can also extend your hands long as your hips become more flexible. Hold for 30 seconds.
- **Malasana/Yogi Squat:** While standing, turn your toes out about 45 degrees, bringing your heels in

towards one another. Bring your hands to prayer at your chest and squat down as you place your elbows inside your inner knees. Press your elbows into your knees to lengthen your spine. You may sway side to side or hold still. If this is intense, you can place a block or folded towel beneath your sacrum to prop you up. Hold for 30 seconds.

- **Gentle Backbends:** Maintaining a flexible spine is essential for overall well-being. Learn how to safely perform gentle backbends while seated, which help to counteract the effects of prolonged sitting, improve posture, and keep your spine supple.

This exercise is great for seniors and those experiencing back pain.

To do this exercise:

- Sit in a comfortable position with your hands on your lower back, fingers facing down, and thumbs around your hips toward you.

- Gently arch your back, feeling the stretch through your spine. Hold for 5-10 seconds.
- Release and repeat 2-3 times.

As you practice these flexibility-enhancing poses, remember to prioritize your breath and listen to your body. Flexibility improves gradually over time, so be patient with yourself and avoid pushing too hard. The journey toward greater flexibility is about self-care, self-acceptance, and nurturing your body's unique abilities.

In the upcoming chapters, you'll explore chair yoga for strength, balance, relaxation, and meditation. Each aspect of chair yoga contributes to your holistic well-being, offering you a balanced and adaptable practice that can be tailored to suit your needs and preferences.

6. Chair Yoga for Strength

Strength is the foundation of movement and independence, and chair yoga offers a gentle yet effective way to build and maintain strength. In this chapter, you'll explore a series of chair yoga poses designed to strengthen various muscle groups, promoting stability and vitality in your body.

Leg and Thigh Strengthening Exercises

Discover chair yoga poses that target your legs and thighs. These movements engage your quadriceps, hamstrings, and calf muscles, promoting lower body strength and stability. Strong legs are essential for everyday activities and maintaining mobility as you age.

Core Strengthening Techniques

A strong core supports your spine, improves posture, and enhances balance. Explore chair yoga exercises that engage your core muscles, including your abdominals and lower back. These movements not only strengthen your core but also contribute to better overall body alignment.

Building Arm and Shoulder Strength

Maintaining arm and shoulder strength is important for maintaining your ability to perform everyday tasks with ease. Learn chair yoga poses that work your arms, shoulders, and upper back. These exercises promote upper body strength and flexibility, enhancing your functional fitness.

As you engage in these strength-building poses, remember that chair yoga emphasizes gentle and mindful movements. Focus on your breath and your body's sensations as you work through each pose. Consistent practice over time can lead to improved muscle tone, balance, and overall strength.

In the upcoming chapters, you'll explore chair yoga for balance, relaxation, and meditation. By incorporating each aspect of chair yoga into your routine, you'll create a well-rounded practice that supports your physical and mental well-being.

7. Balance and Stability

Maintaining good balance is essential for preventing falls and maintaining independence, especially as we age. This chapter introduces chair yoga poses that focus on enhancing your balance and stability. By practicing these poses regularly, you'll improve your proprioception, strengthen supporting muscles, and boost your confidence in everyday movements.

One-Legged Poses

Explore chair yoga variations of one-legged poses that challenge your balance and help strengthen the muscles responsible for stability. These poses also promote better alignment, which is crucial for maintaining good posture.

How to perform one-legged chair pose

Begin by taking an Awkward Chair Pose (Utkatasana)

- Stand straight with your feet together and both arms at your sides.
- Slightly bend your knees, so that your thighs become parallel to the floor.
- Your thighs should be low, and your entire body weight should be on your heels.
- Hold both your hands together in a prayer position or Anjali Mudra, and keep them near your heart.
- Keeping your right foot grounded on the floor, start to lift your left foot off the ground.
- Make sure to keep your right knee bent as you cross your left ankle over your right thigh above your knee. Flex your left foot.
- Look down, and you'll see a triangle shape created by your legs.
- Hold this posture for a few breaths.
- Slowly come out of the posture, and return to an upright position.

Release your left leg to the floor, and breathe easily in the one-legged chair pose before switching your legs.

Seated Balancing Exercises

You don't need to stand to work on your balance. Discover a series of seated balancing exercises that engage your core and challenge your equilibrium while seated in the chair. These exercises are suitable for individuals with varying degrees of mobility.

Here are 3 seated balance exercises for seniors that are safe and easily done without leaving your favorite chair.

1. Sit to Stand Squats:
- Stand with or without the support of your hands.
- All your weight should be on your heels.
- Stand straight with your chest upright.
- Lower yourself into a squat position.

- Sit down again.
- Repeat 8-10 times.

2. Bicep Curls

You will need: A sturdy chair (optional) and light weights (if weights are not available, you can use bottles filled with water, or even canned goods will do).

Get set:

- Sit or stand by the chair.

(If sitting) Feet firmly on the ground and hip-width apart.

(If standing) Stand straight with feet hip-width apart.

- Shoulders straight.
- Arms by your sides.

Start:

- Hold the weights in both hands.
- Raise your hands in a vertical motion, up to your shoulders, keeping the wrists straight, and inhale.
- Bring your hands down and exhale. (You can do this one hand at a time too).
- Repeat 8-10 times.

3. Shift Weight Side to Side

You will need: A comfortable chair.

Get set:

Sit keeping your spine straight.

Feet firmly on the ground, hip-width apart.

Start:

- Lean the upper body gently to the right, lift your left hip, keeping feet firmly on the ground. Hold for a count of 5-10.
- Come back to the starting position.
- Repeat leaning to the left side, lifting your right hip.
- Repeat 8-10 sets.

Tips for Improving Stability

In addition to practicing specific poses, this chapter offers tips and techniques to enhance your overall stability. You'll learn about the importance of engaging your core, maintaining a steady gaze, and finding your center of gravity.

Embrace the process and be patient with yourself. Over time, you'll notice increased confidence in your movements and a greater sense of steadiness.

Improving stability in yoga is crucial for maintaining proper alignment, preventing injuries, and deepening your practice. Here are some detailed tips to enhance your stability in various yoga poses:

Mindful Breathing: Focus on your breath as it helps create a stable foundation. Inhale deeply, filling your lungs, and exhale completely, engaging your core muscles gently. This creates a sense of connection between your breath and movement, promoting stability.

Engage Core Muscles: Actively engage your core muscles (transverse abdominis) to provide support to your spine and pelvis. This core engagement stabilizes your body and prevents unnecessary strain on your back.

Alignment Awareness: Pay close attention to proper alignment in each pose. Misaligned joints can lead to instability. Study the alignment cues provided by your instructor, and use props like blocks and straps to assist you in maintaining proper form.

Root Down and Grounding: In standing poses, feel the connection between your feet and the ground. Distribute your weight evenly through your feet, activating the arches and pressing into the four corners of each foot.

Micro-Bend in Joints: Avoid locking out your joints, especially the knees and elbows. Maintain a slight, soft bend to prevent hyperextension and distribute the load more evenly across muscles and ligaments.

Engage Leg Muscles: In standing poses, engage your leg muscles, such as quadriceps and hamstrings, to create stability around your knee joints. This helps in maintaining balance and preventing the knees from collapsing inward or outward.

Shoulder Stability: In poses involving the upper body, like Plank or Downward Dog, draw your shoulder blades down your back and engage your latissimus dorsi muscles. This stabilizes your shoulder girdle and prevents strain on your shoulders and neck.

Gaze Focus: Fix your gaze on a steady point (drishti) to enhance your balance and stability. This also helps calm your mind and improve concentration.

Slow and Controlled Movements: Move slowly and mindfully between poses. This allows you to maintain stability, control, and awareness throughout the transition.

Warm-Up and Preparatory Poses: Begin your practice with gentle warm-up poses that target the muscles and joints you'll engage during more complex poses. Gradually progress to more challenging postures as your body warms up and becomes more stable.

Props Utilization: Don't hesitate to use yoga props like blocks, straps, or bolsters. They provide support and can help you achieve proper alignment, especially if flexibility is a limiting factor.

Progress Gradually: Be patient with yourself. Don't rush into advanced poses before building a strong foundation. Gradually progress as you gain strength, flexibility, and stability.

Balancing Poses: Practice balancing poses to improve stability. Poses like Tree, Warrior III, and Eagle help enhance concentration, core strength, and overall stability.

Practice Regularly: Consistency is key. Regular practice allows your body to adapt, strengthen, and improve stability over time.

Remember, yoga is about self-awareness and growth. Listen to your body, and don't push yourself too hard. Prioritize safety and stability over achieving a specific pose. If you're new to yoga, consider taking classes with a qualified instructor who can provide personalized guidance and adjustments.

In the upcoming chapters, you'll delve into chair yoga for relaxation and meditation, rounding out your practice with mindfulness and stress-relief techniques. By incorporating each aspect of chair yoga into your routine, you're creating a comprehensive approach to your physical and mental well-being.

8. Relaxation and Meditation

In the fast-paced world we live in, finding moments of relaxation and peace is essential for our overall well-being. This chapter introduces you to the calming aspects of chair yoga, focusing on relaxation and meditation techniques that help reduce stress, promote mental clarity, and enhance your sense of inner tranquility.

Deep Breathing Techniques

Learn various deep breathing techniques that can be practiced while seated in a chair. Deep, conscious breathing calms the nervous system, reduces stress, and increases oxygen flow to the body, promoting relaxation and a sense of centeredness.

Here are a couple of deep breathing techniques you can incorporate into your chair yoga practice:

Diaphragmatic Breathing: Sit comfortably in your chair with your spine straight and your hands on your abdomen. Inhale deeply through your nose, allowing your abdomen to rise as you fill your lungs with air. Exhale slowly through your mouth, letting your abdomen fall. Focus on the sensation of your breath and the movement of your abdomen.

4-7-8 Breathing: Sit comfortably and close your eyes. Inhale quietly through your nose for a count of 4. Hold your breath for a count of 7. Exhale slowly through your mouth for a count of 8. Repeat this cycle a few times, gradually increasing the count if comfortable.

Alternate Nostril Breathing: Sit with your spine straight. Using your right thumb, close off your right nostril and inhale deeply through your left nostril. Close your left nostril with your right ring finger, release your right nostril, and exhale through it. Inhale through your right nostril, close it off, release the left nostril, and exhale through it. Continue alternating nostrils as you inhale and exhale.

Remember to always breathe naturally and comfortably; don't force your breath. Deep breathing can help relax your body and mind during chair yoga practice.

Mindfulness and Relaxation while Seated

Discover how to practice mindfulness and relaxation even in a seated position. These techniques involve directing your awareness to your body, sensations, and breath. By being present in the moment, you can alleviate stress and cultivate a sense of inner peace.

Guided Chair Yoga Meditation

Explore guided meditation practices designed specifically for chair yoga. These guided sessions will lead you through visualization, body scan, and mindfulness exercises, allowing you to experience deep relaxation and a connection to your inner self.

Sure, let's get started with a guided chair yoga meditation. Find a comfortable chair and sit with your feet flat on the floor, hands resting on your lap. Close your eyes and take a deep breath in through your nose, and exhale through your mouth. Let's begin:

- **Grounding Breath:** Inhale deeply through your nose, feeling your belly rise. Exhale slowly through your mouth, releasing any tension. Repeat this a few times, focusing solely on your breath.
- **Neck Stretches:** Gently tilt your head to the right, feeling a stretch on the left side of your neck. Hold for a few breaths, then switch to the other side. Keep your breath steady.
- **Shoulder Rolls:** Inhale as you lift your shoulders up towards your ears, and exhale as you roll them back and

down. Repeat this motion a few times, letting go of any shoulder tension.

- **Seated Cat-Cow:** Inhale, arch your back, and lift your chest (cow pose). Exhale, round your spine, and drop your chin to your chest (cat pose). Continue this gentle movement with your breath for a minute.
- **Spinal Twist:** Place your right hand on the outside of your left thigh and gently twist to the left, looking over your left shoulder. Hold for a few breaths, then switch sides.
- **Deep Breathing:** Place your hands on your belly. Inhale deeply through your nose, expanding your belly, and exhale slowly through your mouth, drawing your navel in. Feel your breath nourishing your body.
- **Mindful Awareness:** Bring your attention to each part of your body, starting from your toes and gradually moving up to your head. Notice any sensations or areas of tension.

Breathe into those areas, allowing them to release.

- **Closing:** Gently open your eyes and sit quietly for a moment, feeling the calm energy you've cultivated. When you're ready, slowly stand up and carry this sense of relaxation with you.

Remember, the key is to go at your own pace and listen to your body. This chair yoga meditation can be modified to suit your comfort level and any physical limitations you may have.

As you engage in these relaxation and meditation techniques, remember that the benefits go beyond the practice itself. Regular relaxation and mindfulness can lead to improved sleep, reduced anxiety, and a more positive outlook on life. By incorporating these practices into your chair yoga routine, you're nurturing not only your physical health but also your mental and emotional well-being.

In the following chapters, you'll explore chair yoga routines and adaptations for specific needs, empowering you to tailor your practice to suit your individual goals and circumstances.

9. Chair Yoga Routines

In this chapter, you'll learn how to structure chair yoga routines that cater to different time constraints and needs. Whether you have just a few minutes to spare or want to dedicate a longer session to your practice, these routines provide a framework for a well-rounded chair yoga experience.

15-Minute Daily Chair Yoga Routine

Discover a concise chair yoga routine that you can easily integrate into your daily schedule. This routine includes a selection of poses that focus on flexibility, strength, balance, and relaxation, ensuring that you can maintain your practice even on busy days.

Gentle Morning Chair Sequence

Start your day on a positive note with a chair yoga sequence designed to awaken your body and mind. These gentle movements promote circulation, release tension, and set a peaceful tone for the rest of your day.

Relaxing Evening Chair Sequence

Unwind and prepare for a restful night's sleep with a calming chair yoga routine. This sequence focuses on relaxation, deep breathing, and gentle stretches, helping you release the stresses of the day and ease into a peaceful evening.

These chair yoga routines offer versatility, allowing you to customize your practice based on your energy levels and goals. Remember, consistency is key, so even short and focused routines can have a significant impact on your overall well-being.

In the upcoming chapter, you'll explore adaptations of chair yoga for specific needs and abilities, providing you with the tools to make your practice accessible and effective for your unique circumstances.

10. Adapting Chair Yoga

Adapting chair yoga to cater to various needs and abilities is a testament to its inclusive nature. In this chapter, you'll explore modifications and variations that ensure everyone can benefit from chair yoga, regardless of their physical condition or limitations.

Chair Yoga for Seniors with Limited Mobility

Learn how to tailor chair yoga poses for seniors with limited mobility. Discover seated poses that provide gentle stretches and movements to maintain joint health, improve circulation, and enhance flexibility, all while accommodating varying levels of mobility.

Chair Yoga for Joint Pain Relief

If you're dealing with joint pain, chair yoga can offer relief without exacerbating discomfort. This section provides poses and techniques to ease joint pain, focusing on gentle movements that support joint health and minimize strain.

Chair Yoga Modifications for Different Abilities

Every individual's body is unique, and chair yoga can be adapted to suit diverse abilities. Explore modifications for poses that cater to both beginners and those with more advanced yoga experience. Learn how to use props effectively to create a safe and comfortable practice.

By understanding how to adapt chair yoga to your specific needs, you're embracing the true spirit of the practice, one that values self-care, self-acceptance, and individuality. As you incorporate these adaptations into your routine, you'll find that chair yoga becomes a tool for empowerment and well-being, regardless of your circumstances.

In the next chapter, you'll find tips for integrating chair yoga into your daily life and resources for further learning. This marks the culmination of your chair yoga journey, providing you with the tools to continue cultivating physical and mental well-being through this enriching practice.

11. Integrating Chair Yoga into Daily Life

Bringing the benefits of chair yoga beyond the mat and into your daily routine can lead to lasting improvements in your overall well-being. In this chapter, you'll discover practical ways to seamlessly incorporate chair yoga into different aspects of your life, from morning to evening.

Incorporating Chair Yoga into Morning and Bedtime Routines

Start your day with intention by adding a few minutes of chair yoga to your morning routine. These gentle movements can help you awaken your body, increase circulation, and set a positive tone for the day ahead. Likewise, integrating chair yoga into your bedtime routine can promote relaxation and better sleep quality.

Using Chair Yoga for Stress Relief

Life's demands can often lead to stress and tension. Learn how chair yoga can become your go-to tool for managing stress. Explore breathing techniques and calming poses that can be practiced even in the midst of a busy day, offering you moments of respite and tranquility.

Chair Yoga in Social Settings

Chair yoga is not limited to solitary practice; it can also be a wonderful way to connect with others. Discover how to incorporate chair yoga into social gatherings, whether it's a family reunion, community event, or a friendly get-together. Share the benefits of chair yoga with others and create a sense of unity through movement and mindfulness.

By weaving chair yoga into your daily life, you're ensuring that its positive impact becomes an integral part of your routine. As you explore the various ways to integrate chair yoga, you're embracing a holistic approach to well-being that extends far beyond the physical aspects of the practice.

In the final chapter, you'll find answers to frequently asked questions, addressing common concerns and offering troubleshooting tips. This comprehensive guide is designed to equip you with the knowledge and tools you need to continue your chair yoga journey with confidence.

12. Conclusion

Congratulations on completing your journey through "Chair Yoga for Seniors." This concluding chapter serves as a reflection on your experience and a reminder of the valuable insights you've gained on your path to improved physical and mental well-being.

Your Chair Yoga Journey

Take a moment to reflect on how far you've come since the beginning of this book. From understanding the foundations of chair yoga to practicing poses, relaxation techniques, and mindfulness, you've embarked on a transformative journey that has the potential to enhance your quality of life.

Resources for Further Learning

As you continue your chair yoga practice, you might want to explore further resources to deepen your understanding and skills.

This chapter provides recommendations for books, online tutorials, and local classes that can support your ongoing journey.

Here are some resources to help you further your learning of chair yoga:

- **YouTube:** Search for chair yoga tutorials on platforms like YouTube. Many instructors offer free videos that guide you through various chair yoga poses and routines.
- **Online Courses:** Websites like Udemy, Coursera, and Skillshare might have online courses specifically dedicated to chair yoga. These courses could offer more structured learning experiences.
- **Books:** Look for books on chair yoga at your local bookstore or online retailers.
- **Apps:** Check if there are any apps available on app stores that provide chair yoga routines and instructions.

Apps can be a convenient way to practice on-the-go.

- **Local Classes:** Search for local fitness centers, community centers, or senior centers that might offer chair yoga classes. In-person instruction can provide personalized guidance.
- **Online Communities:** Join online forums or social media groups focused on yoga. You can ask for recommendations and tips from experienced practitioners.
- **Yoga Studios:** Some yoga studios offer specialized chair yoga classes. If you're comfortable attending in-person sessions, this could be a great way to learn from an instructor.

Embracing a Lifelong Practice

Chair yoga is not just a short-term endeavor; it's a practice that can bring benefits throughout your life. As you incorporate chair yoga into your routine, remember that the journey is ongoing. The poses and techniques you've learned are tools you can carry with you to promote well-being, relaxation, and self-care in any situation.

Acknowledgments

A special acknowledgement goes to all those who supported you on your chair yoga journey from friends and family to teachers and fellow practitioners. Your dedication to your practice and your commitment to self-improvement are commendable.

With this conclusion, you're equipped to continue your chair yoga practice with confidence and purpose. May the lessons and techniques you've gained from this book serve as a foundation for a healthier, more balanced, and fulfilling life. As you carry the benefits of chair yoga into your future, remember that every breath, movement, and moment of mindfulness contributes to your well-being.

Scan here for more books Dr James Fredrick

Other Books Written by Dr James Fredrick

- **Stop Overthinking**
- **Mexico Travel Guide**
- **Spain Travel Guide**
- **Paris Travel Guide**